Hyperpigmentation Cure Guide Book

Secrets to Smoothen uneven Skin

By

Talia Andrus

Table of Contents

Introduction

In the bustling city of Radiantville, a young artist named Mia had a dream to share her creativity with the world. But there was one thing holding her back: hyperpigmentation. Dark spots on her face had become her constant companion, making her feel self-conscious and overshadowing her artistic brilliance.

One day, while strolling through the city's enchanting park, Mia met an enigmatic woman named Luna. Luna had an otherworldly glow, and she seemed to radiate confidence. Intrigued, Mia shared her struggles with hyperpigmentation.

Luna smiled warmly and revealed a secret potion she had concocted, handed down through generations in her family. The magical serum was said to fade away dark spots and bring out the skin's natural luminosity. Eager to embrace her true self, Mia decided to give it a try.

Over the next few weeks, Mia diligently applied the serum, and to her amazement, her hyperpigmentation started fading away. As her skin began to glow, so did her confidence. Emboldened by this newfound transformation, Mia unveiled her stunning art collection at a local gallery.

To her delight, the artworks resonated with people, captivating their hearts and minds. Word spread like wildfire, and soon Mia's art became a sensation, drawing admirers from far and wide. Her story of overcoming hyperpigmentation and embracing her true self inspired countless others, giving them the courage to pursue their dreams.

As Mia's fame grew, she didn't forget Luna's kindness. Grateful for the magical serum that had changed her life, she started a charity to help others with skin concerns feel confident in their own skin. The "Radiant Hearts Foundation" became a beacon of hope for those struggling with hyperpigmentation, offering support and skincare solutions to all.

In the end, Mia's journey from self-doubt to empowerment taught her that true beauty shines from within. Embracing her uniqueness and celebrating her skin's journey became a testament to her resilience and creativity. And so, in the vibrant city of Radiantville, the tale of Mia's radiant transformation became a legend, inspiring generations to come.

Chapter 1

Concepts on hyperpigmentation

Hyperpigmentation and uneven skin tone are common skin concerns that affect people of all ages and skin types. Understanding the concept behind these conditions can help individuals take appropriate measures to address and manage them effectively.

Hyperpigmentation
Hyperpigmentation refers to the darkening or discoloration of certain areas of the skin due to an overproduction of melanin, the pigment responsible for the color of our skin, hair, and eyes. When there is an excessive amount of melanin in specific areas, it leads to the formation of darker patches, spots, or patches on the skin.The

following are the most prevalent kinds of hyperpigmentation; Sunspots or Solar Lentigines; These are caused by sun exposure and are often seen in areas exposed to the sun, such as the face, hands, arms, and shoulders.

Types of Hyperpigmentation

Melasma: This type of hyperpigmentation is characterized by larger and irregular patches, usually appearing on the cheeks, forehead, upper lip, and chin. Hormonal changes, such as pregnancy or birth control pill use, can trigger melasma.

Post-Inflammatory Hyperpigmentation (PIH): PIH occurs after skin inflammation or injury, like acne, eczema, or a wound. It leaves behind dark spots or marks as the skin heals.

Aspect of Hyperpigmentation

Uneven Skin Tone

Uneven skin tone refers to the irregular distribution of color across the skin's surface, resulting in areas of varying shades and tones. It can be caused by multiple factors, including hyperpigmentation, sun damage, environmental exposure, genetics, and aging. Uneven skin tone may manifest as:

Dark Spots

As discussed earlier, hyperpigmentation leads to the appearance of dark spots or patches on the skin, contributing to uneven skin tone.

Redness

Skin conditions like rosacea or excessive sun exposure can cause redness, making the skin tone appear uneven.

Dullness

A lack of radiance or glow can make the skin look lackluster and uneven.

Addressing Hyperpigmentation and Uneven Skin Tone

Sun Protection

Regularly applying a broad-spectrum sunscreen with a high SPF is crucial to preventing further hyperpigmentation and uneven skin tone caused by sun exposure.

Skincare Products

Using skincare products containing active ingredients like niacinamide, alpha arbutin, vitamin C, and retinol can help reduce hyperpigmentation, even out the skin tone, and improve skin texture.

Exfoliation

Gentle exfoliation with chemical exfoliants like alpha hydroxy acids (AHAs) or beta hydroxy acids (BHAs) can aid in removing dead skin cells, promoting cell turnover, and improving skin tone.

Professional Treatments

For severe hyperpigmentation, seeking professional treatments like chemical peels, laser therapy, or microdermabrasion may be beneficial.

Consistent Skincare Routine

Establishing a consistent skincare routine tailored to your skin type and concerns is essential for achieving and maintaining an even skin tone.

Lifestyle Habits

Adopting a healthy lifestyle, including a balanced diet, regular exercise, adequate hydration, and stress management, can positively impact skin health.

The key is Patience

It's important to note that treating hyperpigmentation and uneven skin tone requires patience, as visible results may take time. If the conditions persist or worsen, consulting a dermatologist or skincare professional is recommended to develop a personalized treatment plan.

Chapter 2

Prevention of Hyperpigmentation and Uneven Skin Tone

Avoid Skin Irritants
Certain skincare products or harsh chemicals can trigger inflammation and worsen hyperpigmentation. Opt for gentle, non-comedogenic products that suit your skin type.

Use Sun-Protective Clothing When spending extended periods outdoors, wear wide-brimmed hats, long sleeves, and sunglasses to shield your skin from harmful UV rays.

Manage Hormonal Changes

If you're experiencing hormonal fluctuations due to pregnancy, menopause, or birth control, consult with a healthcare professional to manage the effects on your skin.

Be Cautious with Hair Removal

Procedures like waxing and laser hair removal can cause skin irritation and lead to post-inflammatory hyperpigmentation. If prone to such reactions, consider alternative hair removal methods.

Gentle Cleansing

Use a mild, soap-free cleanser to cleanse your face twice daily, and avoid scrubbing the skin vigorously, as it may worsen pigmentation issues.

Balanced Diet: To maintain skin health, eat a diet high in antioxidants, vitamins, and minerals. Fruits, vegetables, nuts, and fish can all help to maintain a healthy complexion.

Stress Management

Chronic stress can aggravate skin conditions, including hyperpigmentation. Practice stress-reduction techniques like meditation, yoga, or deep breathing to promote overall well-being.

Maintaining an Even Skin Tone

Moisturize

Regularly moisturize your skin to maintain hydration and a smooth texture. Hydrated skin appears healthier and more even in tone.

Avoid Irritants

Steer clear of skincare products or makeup that may cause irritation or allergic reactions, as they can contribute to uneven skin tone.

Regular Exfoliation

Exfoliate gently once or twice a week to remove dead skin cells and reveal a brighter, more even complexion.

Stay Hydrated

Drink plenty of water to maintain skin hydration and promote a radiant appearance.

Sleep Well

Adequate sleep is essential for skin repair and rejuvenation. Attempt to get 7-9 hours of sleep per night.

Professional Advice

If you have persistent concerns with hyperpigmentation or uneven skin tone, consult a dermatologist or skincare professional. They can make customised recommendations and treatments based on your specific requirements.

Remember that individual responses to skincare products and treatments may vary. It's essential to be patient and consistent with your skincare routine and make lifestyle changes to support overall skin health. By adopting a preventive approach and using appropriate treatments, you can work towards achieving and maintaining a more even and radiant complexion.

Chapter 3

Treatment products for Hyperpigmentation

HyperClear Hyperpigmentation Serum

HyperClear Hyperpigmentation Serum is a powerful skincare product specifically designed to target and treat hyperpigmentation issues. Hyperpigmentation is a common skin condition characterized by the darkening of certain areas of the skin due to an overproduction of melanin, which can be caused by factors such as sun exposure, hormonal changes, inflammation, and acne scarring.

Key Ingredients

Niacinamide: This ingredient is a form of vitamin B3 and is known for its ability to regulate the production of melanin, effectively reducing the appearance of dark spots and uneven skin tone.

Alpha Arbutin: Derived from the bearberry plant, alpha arbutin works as a natural skin brightener and is effective in reducing the appearance of dark spots and discolorations.

Licorice Root Extract: This natural ingredient contains glabridin, which inhibits the enzyme responsible for melanin production, helping to fade dark spots and brighten the skin.

Vitamin C: As an antioxidant, vitamin C helps protect the skin from free radicals and aids in collagen production, promoting a more even skin tone and reducing hyperpigmentation.

Retinol: A derivative of vitamin A, retinol accelerates cell turnover and enhances collagen production, effectively fading dark spots and revealing a brighter complexion.

Hyaluronic Acid: This ingredient hydrates and plumps the skin, improving its overall texture and appearance.

How to Use:

Cleanse your face thoroughly before application.

Apply a small amount of the HyperClear Hyperpigmentation Serum to the affected areas.

Use the product twice daily, in the morning and evening, for best results.

Follow up with a broad-spectrum sunscreen during the day to protect your skin from further hyperpigmentation caused by sun exposure.

HyperClear Hyperpigmentation Serum offers several benefits

Reduces Dark Spots

The powerful combination of ingredients helps fade dark spots, sunspots, and acne scars, leading to a more even skin tone.

Brightens Complexion

By inhibiting melanin production, the serum helps to brighten and illuminate the skin, giving it a radiant and healthy appearance.

Improves Texture

Regular use of the serum promotes skin cell turnover, which results in smoother and more refined skin texture.

Hydrates the Skin

The inclusion of hyaluronic acid ensures the skin remains hydrated and plump, reducing the appearance of fine lines and wrinkles.

Promotes Even Skin Tone

With consistent use, the serum helps to even out the skin tone, reducing the appearance of blotchiness and discolorations.

Enhances Skin Clarity

HyperClear Hyperpigmentation Serum works to clarify the complexion, giving the skin a more luminous and youthful glow.

Addresses Age Spots

The potent combination of active ingredients targets age spots and sunspots, gradually fading their appearance over time.

Non-Greasy Formula

The lightweight and non-greasy formula of the serum make it easily absorbed by the skin, making it suitable for use under makeup and other skincare products.

Boosts Confidence

As hyperpigmentation issues are addressed, the overall improvement in skin appearance can boost self-confidence and promote a positive body image.

Suitable for All Skin Types
The formulation is gentle and suitable for all skin types, including sensitive skin.

Potential Side Effects

While HyperClear Hyperpigmentation Serum is generally well-tolerated by most individuals, it's essential to be aware of potential side effects:

Skin Sensitivity
Some users may experience mild irritation, redness, or itching, especially during the initial stages of use.

Sun Sensitivity

As the skin is more vulnerable to sun damage during hyperpigmentation treatment, it's crucial to wear sunscreen daily and limit sun exposure to prevent further darkening of the affected areas.

Retinol Sensitivity

Individuals new to retinol might experience initial dryness or peeling. Gradually introduce the product into your skincare routine to minimize potential side effects.

Allergic Reactions

While rare, some individuals may be sensitive to specific ingredients in the serum. Conduct a patch test before applying the product to your entire face.

Precautions

Patience is Key

Hyperpigmentation treatment can take time to show noticeable results. Consistent use over several weeks is necessary to see a significant improvement in skin tone.

Gradual Incorporation

If you're new to using active skincare ingredients like retinol or alpha arbutin, start by applying the serum every other day to allow your skin to adjust.

Avoid Eye Area

When applying the serum, avoid the delicate eye area, as some ingredients may cause irritation or sensitivity.

Use with Caution During Pregnancy

If you are pregnant or breastfeeding, consult your healthcare professional

before using the product, as some
ingredients may not be recommended
during this period.

Chapter 4

Other products that can be used to help prevent hyperpigmentation

Vitamin C Serum

Vitamin C is an antioxidant that helps brighten the skin and inhibit melanin production, which can prevent dark spots and uneven skin tone.

Vitamin C serum is a popular skincare product known for its numerous benefits for the skin. It is formulated with a stable and potent form of vitamin C, usually ascorbic acid or its derivatives, such as L-ascorbic acid, tetrahexyldecyl ascorbate, or magnesium ascorbyl phosphate. The serum is designed to be applied topically to the skin and is available in various concentrations, typically ranging from 5% to 20%.

Benefits of Vitamin C Serum

Antioxidant Properties: Vitamin C is a potent antioxidant that helps neutralize free radicals, which are unstable molecules that can damage skin cells and lead to premature aging. By reducing oxidative stress, vitamin C helps protect the skin from environmental damage caused by pollution, UV rays, and other external aggressors.

Brightening Effect: Vitamin C has skin-brightening properties, as it inhibits the production of melanin, the pigment responsible for dark spots and hyperpigmentation. Regular use of vitamin C serum can help even out skin tone and reduce the appearance of dark spots, acne scars, and sunspots.

Collagen Production: Vitamin C plays a vital role in collagen synthesis, which is crucial for maintaining skin elasticity and firmness. By promoting collagen production, vitamin C helps improve the skin's texture, reducing the appearance of fine lines and wrinkles.

Sun Damage Repair: As an antioxidant, vitamin C helps repair sun-damaged skin by stimulating the skin's natural healing processes and supporting skin regeneration.

UV Protection Enhancement: While vitamin C itself cannot replace sunscreen, studies suggest that it can enhance the effectiveness of sunscreens, offering an extra layer of protection against harmful UV rays.

Tips for Using Vitamin C Serum:

Patch Test: Before applying vitamin C serum all over your face, it's advisable to do a patch test on a small area of skin to check for any allergic reactions or sensitivity.

Proper Application: Apply a few drops of the serum to clean, dry skin after cleansing and toning. Gently massage it into the skin, focusing on areas prone to hyperpigmentation and sun damage.

Store Properly: Vitamin C is sensitive to light and air, so it's essential to store the serum in a dark, opaque bottle and keep it tightly sealed to maintain its potency.

Pair with Sunscreen: For maximum protection against UV-induced hyperpigmentation, always use vitamin C serum in conjunction with a broad-spectrum sunscreen.

Keep in mind that vitamin C serum may not be suitable for everyone, especially those with very sensitive skin. If you experience any adverse reactions or have specific skin concerns, consult a dermatologist before incorporating a vitamin C serum into your skincare routine.

Chapter 5

Niacinamide

Niacinamide, also known as vitamin B3 or nicotinamide, is a water-soluble vitamin that can be found in various food sources and is also commonly used in skincare products for its beneficial effects on the skin.

Source of Niacinamide in Food
Niacinamide is naturally present in many food items. Some of the primary food sources of niacinamide include:

Meat: Chicken, turkey, beef, and pork are good sources of niacinamide.

Fish: Tuna, salmon, and other fish contain niacinamide.

Whole Grains: Foods like brown rice, oats, barley, and wheat provide niacinamide.

Legumes: Peas, lentils, and beans contain niacinamide.

Nuts and Seeds: Sunflower seeds, peanuts, and almonds are sources of niacinamide.

Vegetables: Mushrooms, broccoli, avocados, and sweet potatoes contain niacinamide.

Effects of Niacinamide on Hyperpigmentation:

Niacinamide offers several benefits for the skin, and its effects on hyperpigmentation are particularly notable:

Skin Brightening: Niacinamide helps inhibit the transfer of melanin within skin cells, which can reduce the appearance of dark spots and hyperpigmentation. This leads to a brighter and more even complexion.

Reduces Dark Spots: Niacinamide's ability to regulate melanin production can help fade existing dark spots caused by sun damage, acne, or other forms of hyperpigmentation.

Anti-Inflammatory Properties: Niacinamide has anti-inflammatory effects, which can help soothe and calm irritated skin. Inflammation can exacerbate hyperpigmentation, so reducing it is beneficial for improving skin tone.

Strengthens Skin Barrier: Niacinamide supports the skin's natural barrier function, enhancing its ability to retain moisture and protect against external irritants. A healthy skin barrier contributes to overall skin health, including reducing the risk of hyperpigmentation.

Antioxidant Benefits: Niacinamide is a potent antioxidant that helps neutralize free radicals, protecting the skin from environmental damage and reducing oxidative stress. This can prevent further hyperpigmentation caused by external aggressors.

Compatible with Other Ingredients: Niacinamide is relatively stable and can be combined with other skincare ingredients like vitamin C, retinol, and alpha hydroxy acids without causing significant interactions or irritation.

Using Niacinamide for Hyperpigmentation

Product Selection: Look for skincare products that contain niacinamide, such as serums, creams, or spot treatments, specifically formulated to target hyperpigmentation.

Consistent Use: Apply niacinamide-containing products regularly as part of your skincare routine to see noticeable improvements in hyperpigmentation over time.

Sun Protection: Always use sunscreen with a high SPF when using niacinamide or any other skin-brightening ingredient to protect your skin from further sun damage and hyperpigmentation.

Patch Test: Before incorporating a new product with niacinamide into your routine, do a patch test to check for any allergic reactions or sensitivities.

Other Advice: While niacinamide is generally well-tolerated by most skin types, it's essential to monitor how your skin responds to any new ingredient and consult a dermatologist if you have specific skin concerns or conditions. Niacinamide is a valuable addition to a comprehensive skincare routine aimed at improving hyperpigmentation and achieving a more radiant complexion.

Compatible with Other Ingredients: Niacinamide is relatively stable and can be combined with other skincare ingredients like vitamin C, retinol, and alpha hydroxy acids without causing significant interactions or irritation.

Chapter 6

Retinoids

These derivatives of vitamin A promote cell turnover, helping to fade dark spots and improve overall skin texture.Retinoids are a class of chemical compounds derived from vitamin A. They are highly effective in skincare due to their ability to regulate cell turnover and promote collagen production. Retinoids are available in various forms, including natural sources and synthetic derivatives.

Sources of Retinoids

Retinol: Retinol is a natural form of vitamin A found in animal products, such as liver, eggs, and dairy. It is also commonly used in skincare products for its anti-aging and skin-renewing properties.

Beta-Carotene: Beta-carotene is a precursor to vitamin A and is found in colorful fruits and vegetables, such as carrots, sweet potatoes, spinach, and kale. The body converts beta-carotene into retinol, making it another source of retinoids.

Synthetic Derivatives of Retinoids

Retin-A (Tretinoin): Tretinoin is a prescription retinoid and the most potent form of vitamin A used in skincare. It is commonly prescribed to treat acne, hyperpigmentation, and signs of aging.

Adapalene: Adapalene is another prescription retinoid that is used to treat acne and can also be effective in improving skin texture and reducing hyperpigmentation.

Effects of Retinoids on Hyperpigmentation

Promotes Exfoliation: Retinoids enhance the shedding of dead skin cells and promote cell turnover, helping to remove the top layer of pigmented skin cells. This exfoliating action leads to a reduction in the appearance of hyperpigmentation.

Inhibits Melanin Production: Retinoids can help regulate melanin production by inhibiting the activity of tyrosinase, an enzyme involved in melanin synthesis. This helps to prevent the formation of dark spots and hyperpigmentation.

Encourages Collagen Production: Regular use of retinoids stimulates collagen production, which can improve skin texture, firmness, and overall tone. This can help reduce the visibility of hyperpigmentation and create a more even complexion.

Accelerates Skin Renewal: Retinoids accelerate the skin's natural renewal process, allowing new and healthier skin cells to replace older, pigmented cells. This contributes to a brighter and more even skin tone.

Using Retinoids for Hyperpigmentation

Gradual Introduction: When starting with retinoids, it's crucial to begin with a lower concentration and gradually increase usage to minimize potential skin irritation.

Sun Protection: Since retinoids can increase the skin's sensitivity to the sun, wearing sunscreen daily is essential to protect the skin and prevent further hyperpigmentation.

Moisturize: Retinoids can cause dryness and irritation, so it's essential to use a moisturizer to keep the skin hydrated and help alleviate potential side effects.

Consistency is Key: To see visible improvements in hyperpigmentation, consistent use of retinoids over several weeks or months is necessary.

Consult a Dermatologist: If you have severe hyperpigmentation or specific skin concerns, it's best to consult with a dermatologist for personalized recommendations and guidance on using retinoids. Also, retinoids are a powerful tool in addressing hyperpigmentation and improving overall skin health. However, they may not be suitable for everyone, especially those with sensitive skin. It's essential to use retinoids responsibly and under the guidance of a dermatologist if needed.

Chapter 7

Licorice Extract

Known for its skin brightening properties, licorice extract can help reduce the appearance of hyperpigmentation in modern skincare due to its skin-brightening and anti-inflammatory properties.

Source of Licorice Extract

The active component of licorice extract responsible for its skin benefits is called *Glabridin*. Glabridin is a natural compound found in licorice root that has antioxidant and anti-inflammatory properties. Licorice extract is commonly used in skincare products, particularly those targeting hyperpigmentation, uneven skin tone, and dark spots.

Effects of Licorice Extract on Hyperpigmentation

Skin Brightening: Glabridin inhibits the activity of an enzyme called tyrosinase, which is responsible for melanin production. By reducing tyrosinase activity, licorice extract helps to prevent excess melanin formation, leading to a brighter and more even skin tone.

Hyperpigmentation Reduction: Due to its melanin-inhibiting properties, licorice extract can help reduce the appearance of hyperpigmentation, including dark spots, sunspots, and post-inflammatory hyperpigmentation caused by acne scars.

Anti-Inflammatory Benefits: Licorice extract contains anti-inflammatory compounds that can help soothe and calm irritated skin. Inflammation can exacerbate hyperpigmentation, so reducing inflammation is essential in the treatment of pigmentation issues.

Sun Damage Protection: Licorice extract's antioxidant properties help protect the skin from free radical damage caused by UV rays and environmental pollutants. This can prevent further hyperpigmentation caused by sun exposure.

Gentle on the Skin: Unlike some other skin-brightening agents, licorice extract is generally well-tolerated by most skin types, including sensitive skin. It is considered a milder alternative to certain skin-lightening ingredients, making it suitable for individuals with easily irritated skin.

Using Licorice Extract for Hyperpigmentation

Licorice extract is commonly found in serums, creams, and spot treatments formulated to target hyperpigmentation. When using products with licorice extract, consistency is key to achieving the desired results.

How to apply

Apply as Directed: Follow the product instructions carefully and apply the product to clean, dry skin as part of your skincare routine.

Sunscreen Protection: Since sun exposure can worsen hyperpigmentation, it's crucial to wear sunscreen daily to protect the skin and maximize the benefits of licorice extract.

Patience is Key: Skin brightening and hyperpigmentation reduction usually take time.
Patch Test: Before incorporating a new product with licorice extract into your routine, do a patch test to ensure you don't have any allergic reactions or sensitivities.

As with any skincare ingredient, it's essential to be patient and consistent in your skincare routine. If you have severe hyperpigmentation or concerns about your skin, consider consulting with a dermatologist for personalized advice and treatment options.

Chapter 8

Alpha Hydroxy Acids (AHAs)

AHAs like glycolic acid and lactic acid exfoliate the skin, helping to fade dark spots and reveal a more even complexion.

Alpha Hydroxy Acids (AHAs) are a group of water-soluble acids that are derived from various natural sources. They are widely used in skincare for their exfoliating and skin-renewing properties. The most common AHAs used in skincare products are glycolic acid, lactic acid, mandelic acid, citric acid, and malic acid.

Sources of Alpha Hydroxy Acids

Glycolic Acid: Derived from sugarcane, glycolic acid is the smallest AHA and can penetrate the skin deeply, making it effective for exfoliating and addressing various skin concerns.

Lactic Acid: This AHA is derived from milk, although the lactic acid used in skincare products is often synthetically produced. Lactic acid is milder than glycolic acid and is well-tolerated by most skin types.

Mandelic Acid: Derived from bitter almonds, mandelic acid has larger molecules, which means it penetrates the skin more slowly and is generally gentler on the skin.

Citric Acid: Found naturally in citrus fruits, citric acid is a mild AHA commonly used in skincare products for its exfoliating and antioxidant properties.

Malic Acid: Derived from apples, malic acid has exfoliating properties and can help improve skin texture and appearance.

Effects of Alpha Hydroxy Acids on Hyperpigmentation

Exfoliation: AHAs work by breaking down the bonds between dead skin cells on the skin's surface, promoting exfoliation. This process helps to remove the top layer of dead skin cells, revealing fresher and brighter skin underneath.

Hyperpigmentation Reduction: By promoting exfoliation, AHAs can help fade dark spots and hyperpigmentation over time. As the top layer of pigmented skin cells is shed, the appearance of dark spots and uneven skin tone is reduced.

Enhanced Skin Cell Turnover: AHAs encourage the skin's natural cell turnover process, which can lead to a more even distribution of melanin and a reduction in the appearance of hyperpigmentation.

Stimulates Collagen Production: Regular use of AHAs can stimulate collagen production, which improves skin texture and can help reduce the appearance of fine lines and wrinkles, creating a more even skin surface.

Using Alpha Hydroxy Acids for Hyperpigmentation

When using AHAs to target hyperpigmentation, it's essential to be mindful of the following:

Start Slowly: If you're new to AHAs, start with a lower concentration and gradually increase usage to avoid potential skin irritation.

Sun Protection: AHAs can increase the skin's sensitivity to the sun. Always wear sunscreen with a high SPF when using AHAs to protect your skin from sun damage and prevent further hyperpigmentation.

Patch Test: Before incorporating a new AHA product into your skincare routine, do a patch test to check for any adverse reactions or sensitivity.

Consistency: Consistent use is key to seeing results. Incorporate AHAs into your skincare routine regularly to experience the benefits on

Chapter 9

Conclusion

To draw the curtain, hyperpigmentation is a common skin condition characterized by dark patches on the skin due to excess melanin production. It can be caused by various factors, including sun exposure, hormonal changes, inflammation, and skin injuries. While hyperpigmentation is generally harmless, it can affect one's self-confidence and appearance. However, with proper precautions such as sun protection, gentle skincare, and timely medical advice, it can be effectively managed and prevented. Remember to consult a dermatologist for personalized guidance on treating and maintaining healthy, even-toned skin. By taking proactive measures, individuals can achieve a more radiant complexion and feel more comfortable in their skin.